A WARD POCKET-BOOK FOR
THE NURSE

by Hilda M. Gration

The Nurse's Encyclopaedia and Guide

A WARD POCKET-BOOK
FOR THE NURSE

by **Hilda M. Gration,** SRN, SCM, DN (Lond.)
*Formerly Sister Tutor, Guy's Hospital,
Examiner in Nursing for the General
Nursing Council of England and Wales*

and **Dorothy L. Holland,** SRN, SCM, DN (Lond.)
*Formerly Sister Tutor, Guy's Hospital,
Member of the General Nursing Council
of England and Wales*

revised by
Joan Brotton, SRN
*Clinical Teacher, Guy's Hospital School of Nursing
Examiner, General Nursing Council of England
and Wales*

FABER AND FABER
London and Boston

First published in 1946
by Faber and Faber Limited
3 Queen Square London WC1
Sixth Edition 1965
Reprinted 1967, 1970, 1971, 1972, 1975
Seventh Edition 1978
Phototypeset in VIP Melior by
Western Printing Services Ltd, Bristol
Printed in Great Britain by
Whitstable Litho Ltd, Whitstable, Kent
All rights reserved

British Library Cataloguing in Publication Data

Gration, Hilda Mary
  A Ward pocket-book for the nurse.
  1. Nursing
  I. Title II. Holland, Dorothy Lizzie
  III. Brotton, Joan
  610.73   RT41

ISBN 0—571—04966—4

Introduction

This little book speaks for itself. It is designed to help the nurse with her practical work in the wards. It may be carried in the pocket and used as a book of reference. It does not attempt to give reasons for the various procedures nor does it explain how they should be carried out, but it states the equipment necessary.

When a nurse observes a treatment performed for the first time, she will learn the method and the use of the various requirements.

Publisher's Note

This book has again been revised by Miss Joan Brotton, who has brought it up to date and included new material. All measurements in the new SI units are given. Mrs Audrey Besterman has drawn new illustrations.

Contents

Illustrations of Ward Instruments and Equipment	13
Preparation for Treatment	35
Methods of Sterilization	37
Requirements for Unsterile Treatments and Investigations	40
Requirements for Aseptic Techniques	65
Weights and Measures	84
Dilution of Lotions	89
Pharmacy Act	91
Poisons and Pharmacy Act	93
Latin Abbreviations	95
Food Values	97

Urine Testing	102
Special Tests	107
Incubation Periods of Infectious Diseases	113
Index	115

WARD INSTRUMENTS AND EQUIPMENT

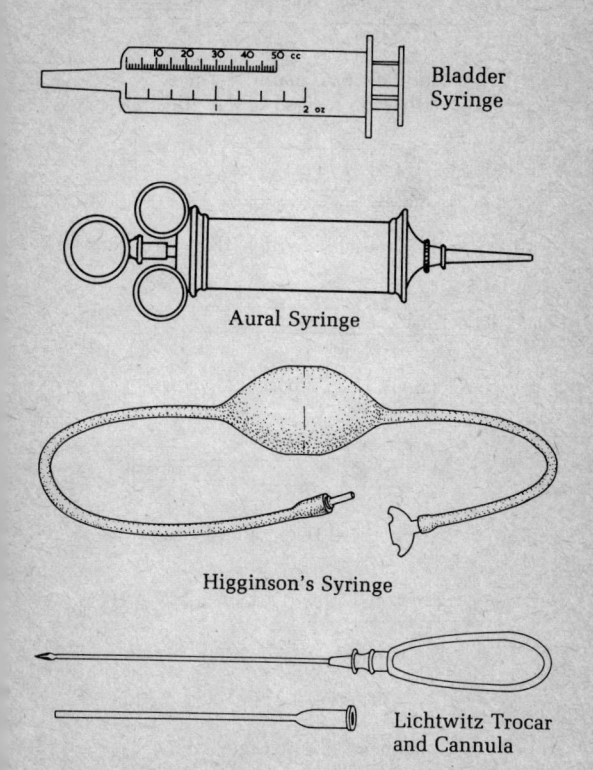

Bladder Syringe

Aural Syringe

Higginson's Syringe

Lichtwitz Trocar and Cannula

Instruments and Equipment

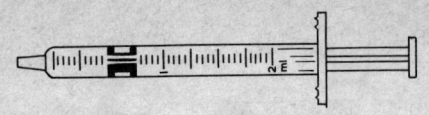

2ml Plastipak Insulin Syringe
Insulin written on reverse side of illustration

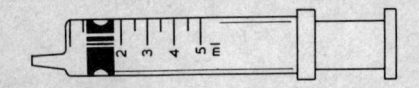

5 ml Steriseal Disposable Syringe (Eccentric Nozzle)

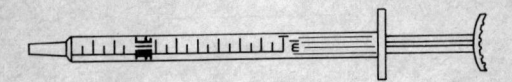

1 ml Gillette Disposable Syringe

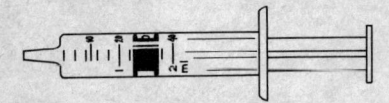

2 ml Steriseal Disposable Syringe

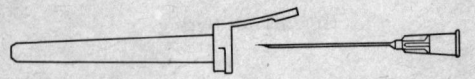

Everett Disposable Hypodermic Needle

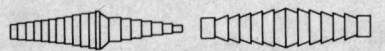

Graduated Plastic Connections

Instruments and Equipment

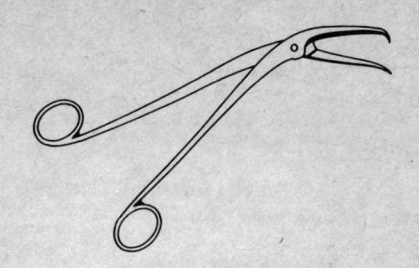

Cheatle's Forceps

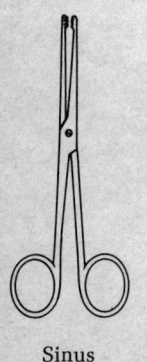

Sinus Forceps

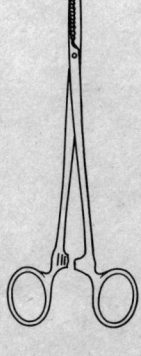

Artery Forceps

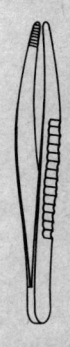

Dressing Forceps

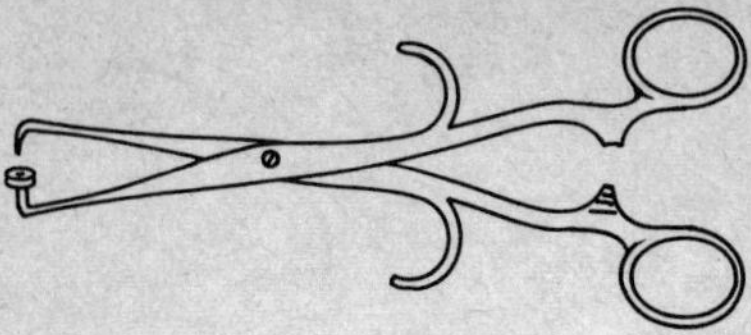

Instruments and Equipment

Tongue Forceps

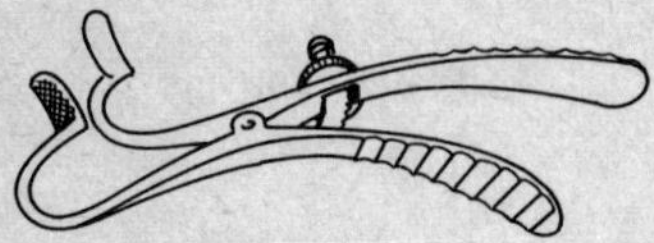

Mouth Gag (Mason's)

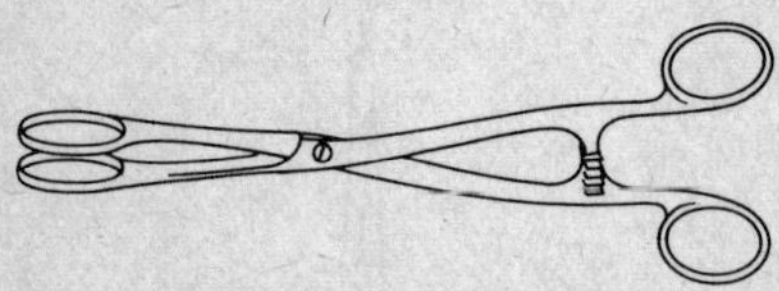

Sponge Holding Forceps

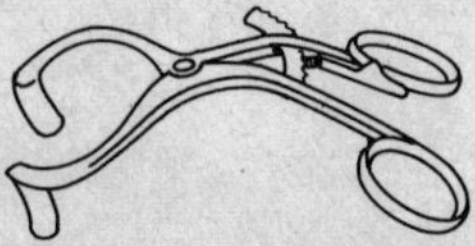

Mouth Gag (Doyen's)

Instruments and Equipment

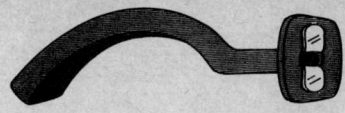

Guedal's Airway

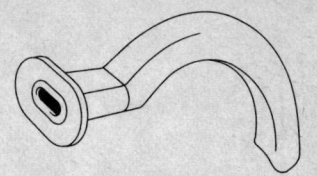

Portex Airway

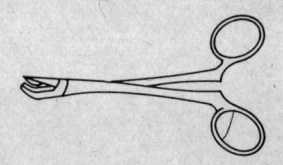

Michel Clip Remover

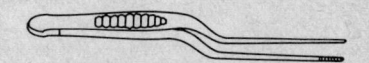

Aural Dressing Forceps

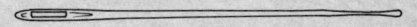

Probe

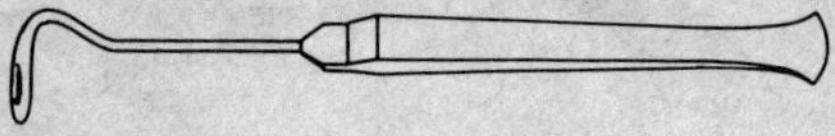

Instruments and Equipment

Aneurysm Needle

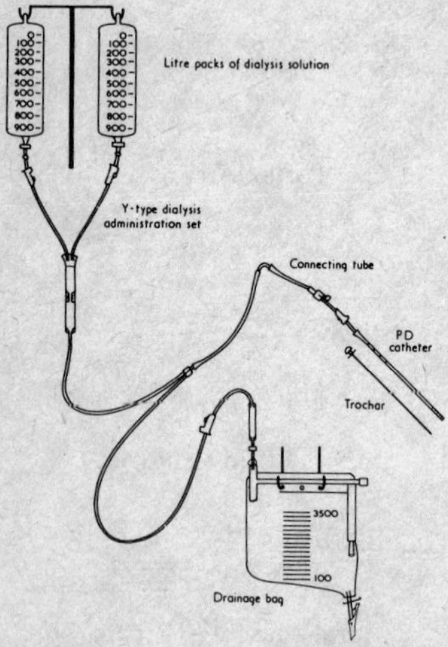

Peritoneal Dialysis Apparatus

- Litre packs of dialysis solution
- Y-type dialysis administration set
- Connecting tube
- P.D catheter
- Trochar
- Drainage bag

Instruments and Equipment

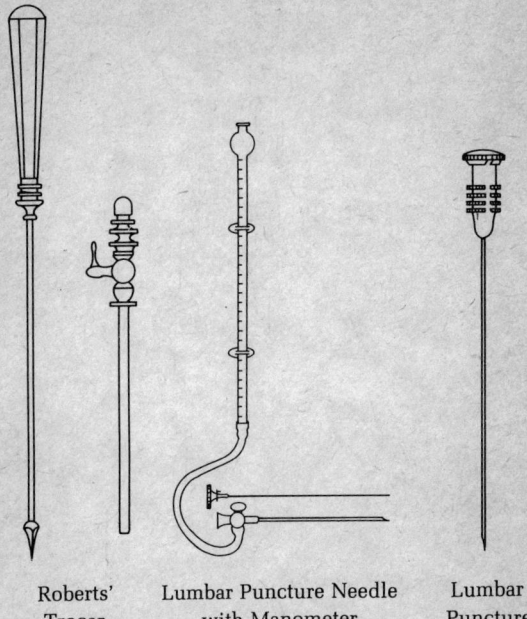

Roberts' Trocar and Cannula

Lumbar Puncture Needle with Manometer

Lumbar Puncture Needle

Instruments and Equipment

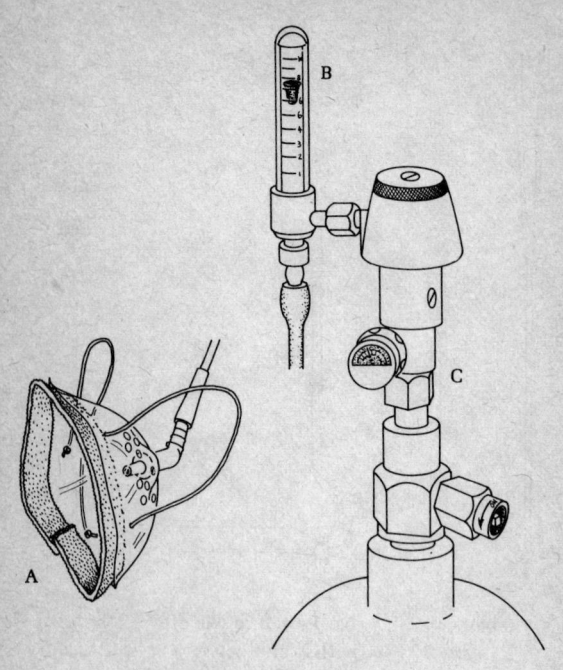

ADMINISTRATION OF OXYGEN

A Disposable M.C. Oxygen Mask
B Flowmeter
C Oxygen cylinder and gauge

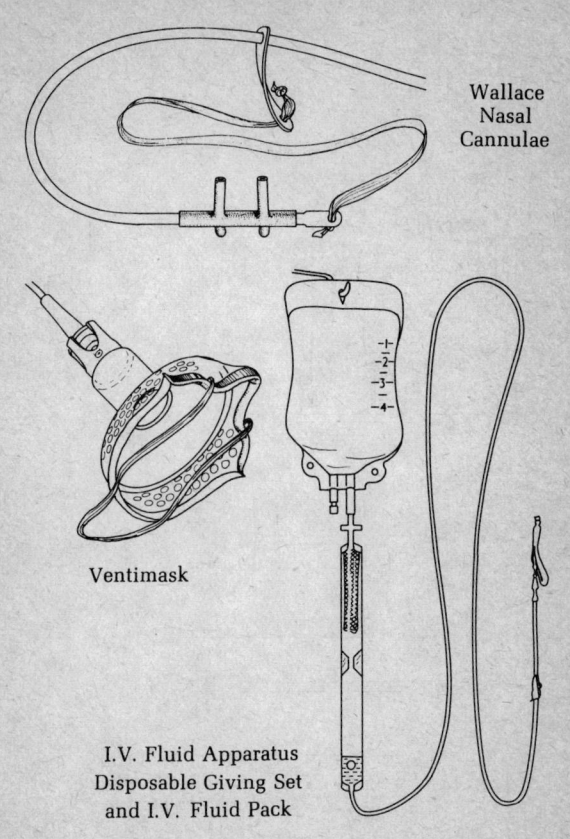

Instruments and Equipment

21

Wallace Nasal Cannulae

Ventimask

I.V. Fluid Apparatus
Disposable Giving Set
and I.V. Fluid Pack

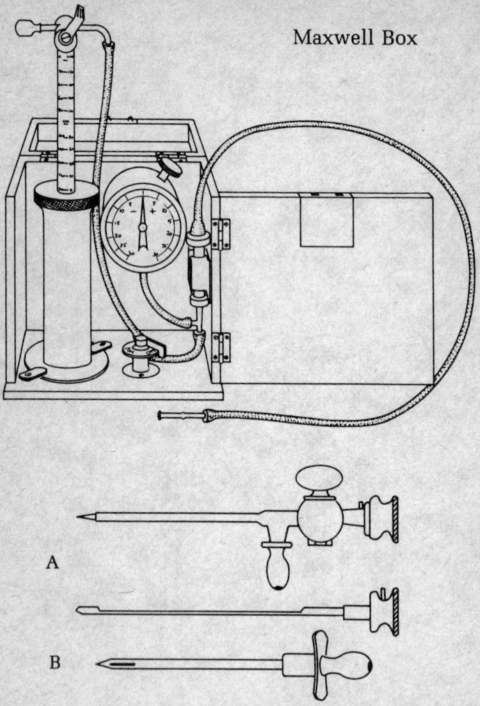

22   Instruments and Equipment

Maxwell Box

APPARATUS FOR ARTIFICIAL PNEUMOTHORAX
A Trocar and cannula for induction. **B** Needle for refill

Instruments and Equipment

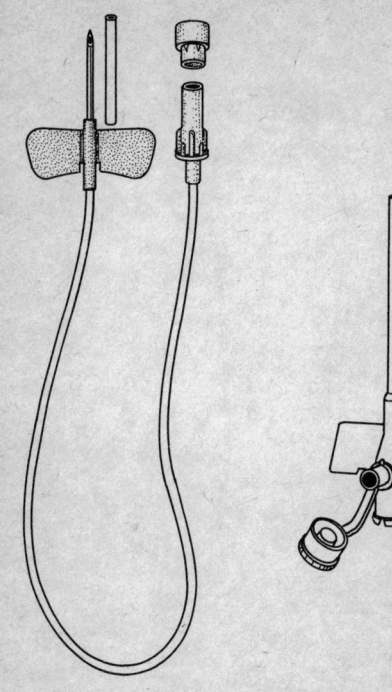

23

Butterfly Cannula

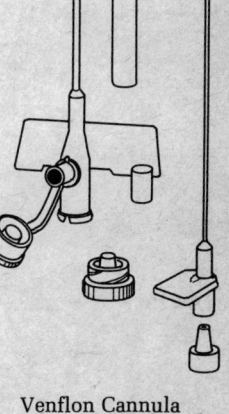

Venflon Cannula

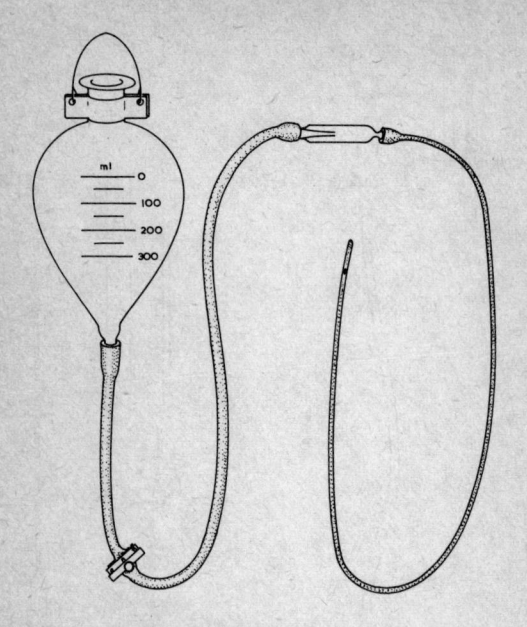

Apparatus for Rectal Infusion

    Burrell's Flask
    Rubber Tubing
    Drip Connection
    Rectal Tube

Instruments and Equipment 25

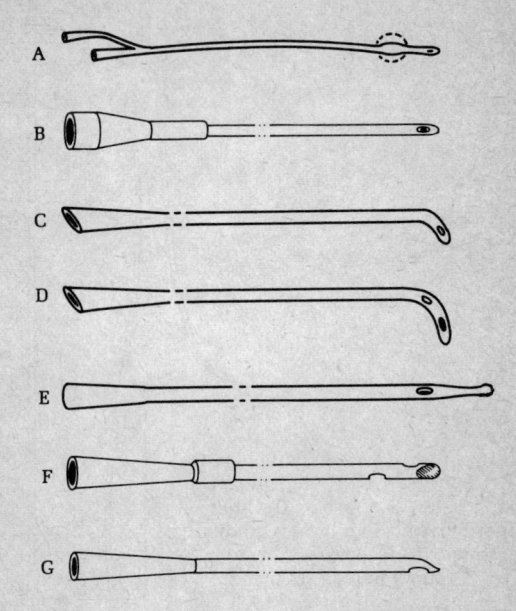

CATHETERS

- **A** Foley
- **B** Disposable Jacques
- **C** Coudé
- **D** Bi-Coudé
- **E** Olive-headed
- **F** Disposable Suction
- **G** Rubber Suction

26   Instruments and Equipment

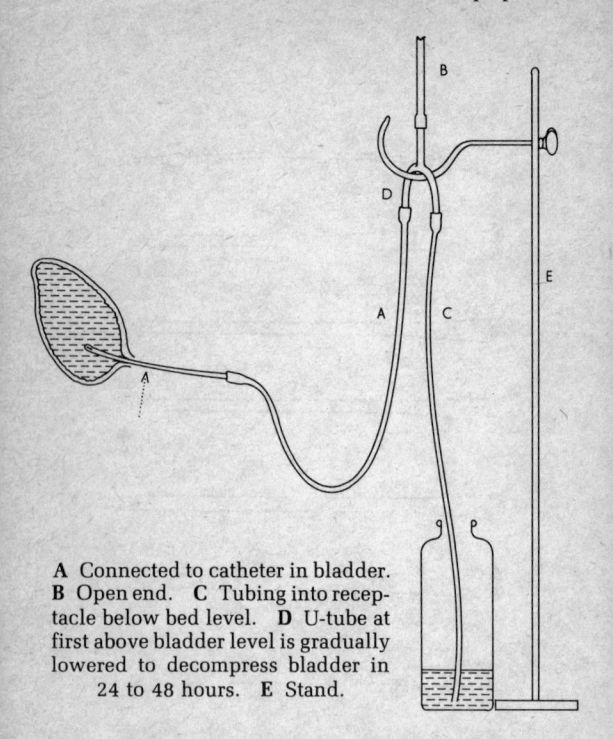

A Connected to catheter in bladder.
B Open end. **C** Tubing into receptacle below bed level. **D** U-tube at first above bladder level is gradually lowered to decompress bladder in 24 to 48 hours. **E** Stand.

APPARATUS FOR GRADUAL DECOMPRESSION OF BLADDER

Instruments and Equipment

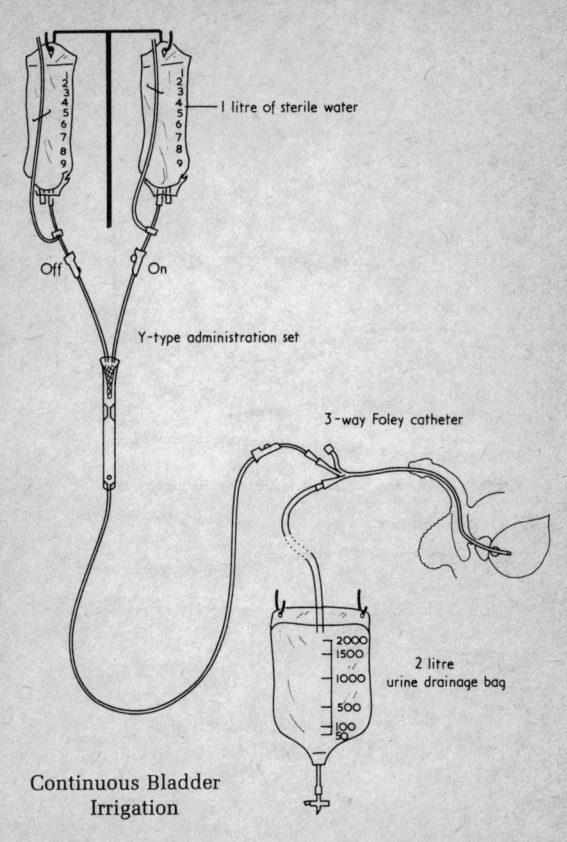

1 litre of sterile water

Off — On

Y-type administration set

3-way Foley catheter

2 litre urine drainage bag

Continuous Bladder Irrigation

28 Instruments and Equipment

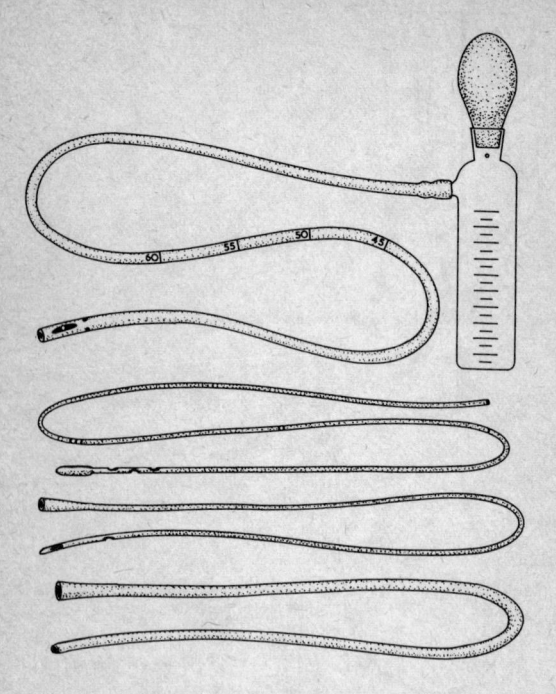

Senoran's Evacuator and Tube
A Ryle's Tube   Oesophageal Tube   Rectal Tube

Instruments and Equipment

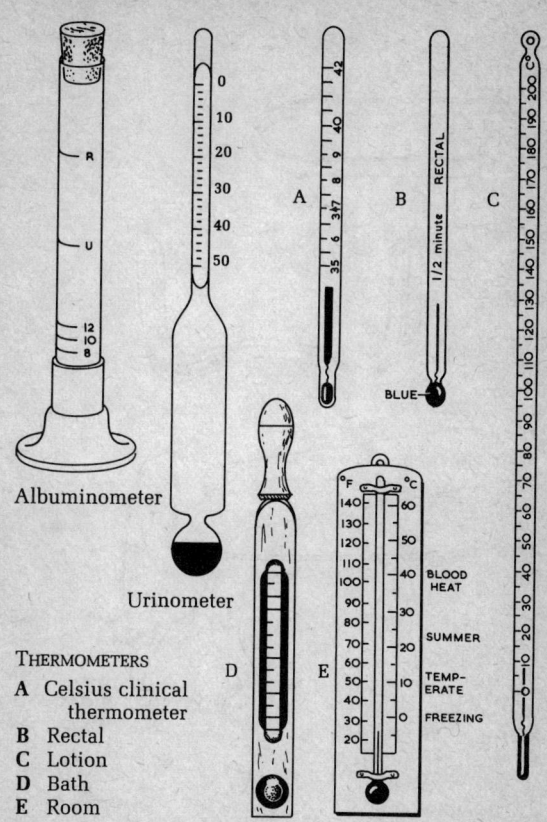

Albuminometer

Urinometer

THERMOMETERS

- **A** Celsius clinical thermometer
- **B** Rectal
- **C** Lotion
- **D** Bath
- **E** Room

Instruments and Equipment

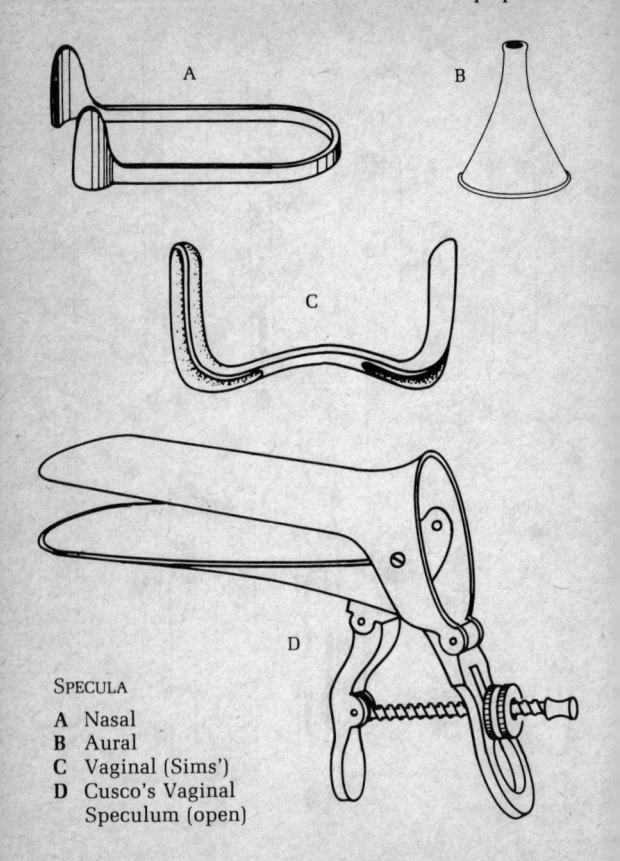

SPECULA

- **A** Nasal
- **B** Aural
- **C** Vaginal (Sims')
- **D** Cusco's Vaginal Speculum (open)

Instruments and Equipment 31

Proctoscope

Apparatus for Vaginal Douche

Hodge's Pessary

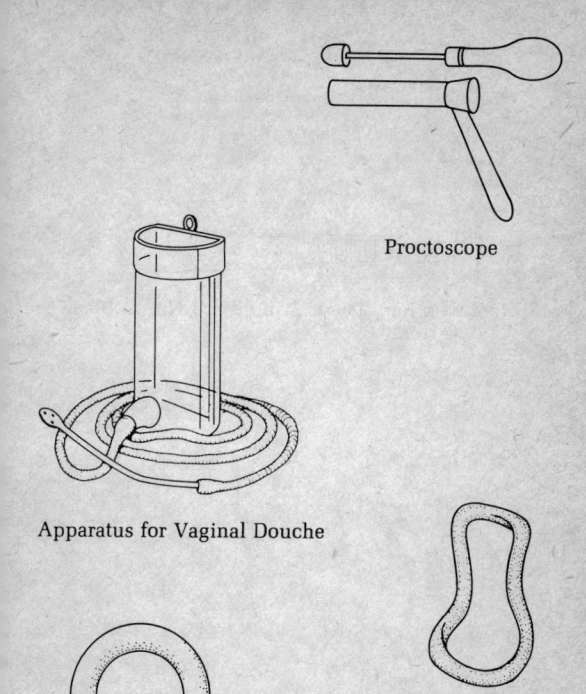

Ring Pessary (P.V.C.)

32 Instruments and Equipment

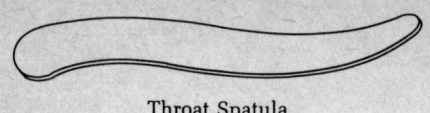

Throat Spatula

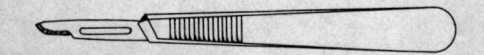

Scalpel with Bard Parker handle and No. 15 Blade

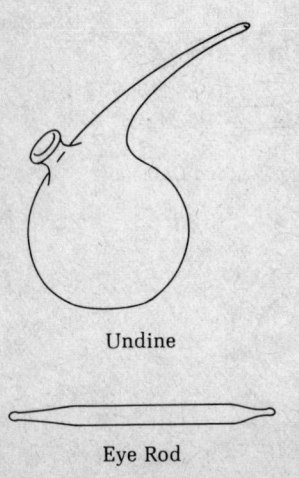

Undine

Eye Rod

Instruments and Equipment

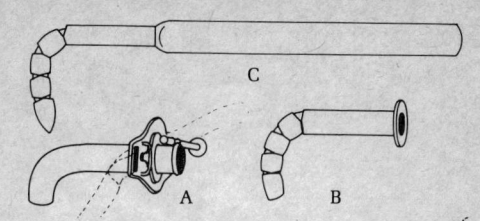

A Outer Tube **B** Inner Tube **C** Introducer
Tracheotomy Tubes (Durham's Lobster-tail)

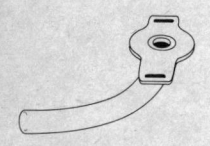

Portex Tracheotomy Tube

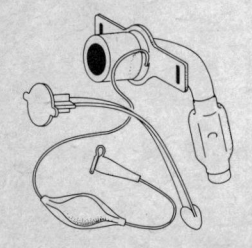

Portex Cuffed Tracheotomy Tube and Introducer

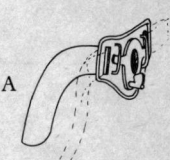

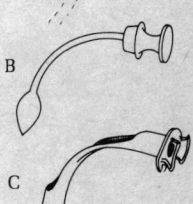

Tracheotomy Tubes (Parker's)

A Outer Tubes
B Introducer
C Inner Tube

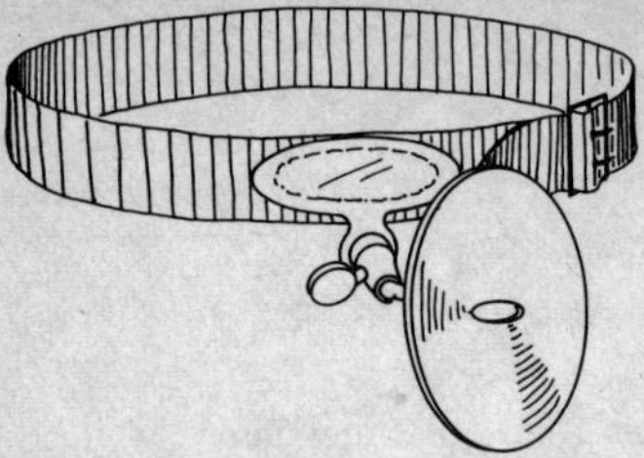

Instruments and Equipment

Head Mirror

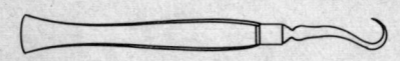

Tracheotomy Hook

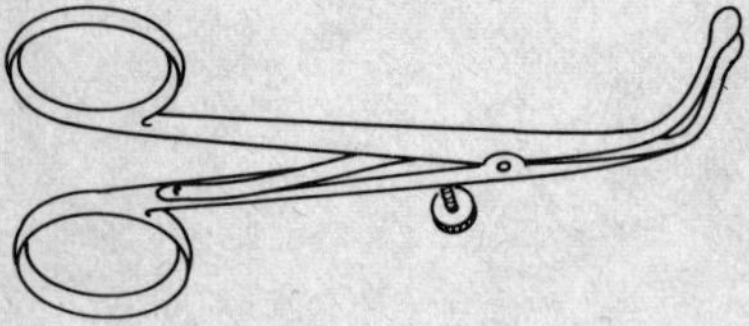

Tracheal Dilator

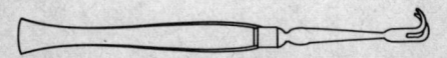

Tracheotomy Retractor

Preparation of a Patient for Treatment

1. When preparing to give any treatment, explain to the patient what is to be done. This is important, for what seems to be a simple routine to the nurse may be alarming to the patient who is nervous and apprehensive.

2. Prepare all requirements to the last detail, so that the treatment can be done in the minimum of time and without having to leave the patient once the procedure has commenced.

3. Close the windows, screen the bed, place the patient in the correct position and cover with a blanket if the bedclothes have been turned back. Throughout the procedure, the nurse must attend to the patient's comfort and carefully observe his general condition. At all times, especially if the treatment is being performed by a doctor, the nurse should watch the reactions of the patient noting any change in colour, pulse and respiration rate, or if he complains of nausea or faintness.

4. Mackintoshes or polythene sheets should be warmed before placing in the bed.

COLLECTING THE APPARATUS

1. Clean the shelves of the trolley and wash any trays to be used.
2. Wool, bandages and adhesive strapping should be placed in an appropriate dish.
3. Collect all requirements methodically, visualizing the procedure and thinking of each item in the order in which it is to be used. This is the best way to ensure nothing is forgotten.
4. Any dish containing sterile equipment should be covered with a lid or second dish.
5. Containers for soiled dressings and instruments should be covered.
6. Masks should be worn for surgical treatments, where there is an open wound, and where there is a possibility of a droplet infection.
7. In the list of requirements, only those described as sterile should be sterilized. All other equipment must be perfectly clean.
8. The nurse's hands are to be washed before and after each treatment and dried with a **clean** towel.

Methods of Sterilization and Disinfection

Prior to disinfection or sterilization all equipment should be thoroughly cleaned. This is usually performed by the Central Sterile Supply Service from where dressings, instruments and other apparatus are sent to the wards and departments in sterile packs.

Sterilization destroys all micro-organisms.

1. *Autoclaves* make use of steam under pressure. With high pressure, high vacuum autoclaves, a pressure of 1.16 Bar or 17 lbs and a temperature of 120° Celsius for 20 minutes, or more commonly 2.18 Bar or 32 lbs pressure at a temperature of 134°C for 3½ minutes is required for sterilization of all types of equipment.

2. *With a low pressure and formaldehyde autoclave* the chamber is under vacuum, with a steam temperature of 70°–80°C. Formaldehyde gas is released into the steam, the amount being related

to the size of the chamber. The time cycle for sterilization is 2 hours.

This method has the advantage in the sterilization of heat labile equipment.

3. *Infra-red chambers* are used mainly for the sterilization of glass. The temperature in the chamber is raised to 180°C and maintained for 10 minutes.

4. *Ethylene oxide chambers* are used mainly for heat labile materials such as plastic, rubber, gum elastic and endoscopes. 10 per cent ethylene oxide gas is pumped into the chamber. The sterilizing time is variable, usually 1–10 hours at a temperature of 60°C and with a high humidity content.

METHODS OF DISINFECTION

Disinfection destroys vegetative pathogens and should only be used as an emergency measure.

1. Chemical Disinfection

    Hycolin 2 per cent
    Hibitane 5 per cent in 70 per cent spirit
    Glutaraldehyde (Cidex) 2 per cent
Immerse equipment for at least 10 minutes

Methods of Sterilization

Glutaraldehyde is unstable after 2 weeks and should be discarded. After chemical disinfection items should be rinsed in sterile distilled water.

2. Heat Disinfection

Boiling. The water in the disinfector should be boiling and items placed below the level of the water line. Boil for 5 minutes.

Pasteurization. This method is usually used for endoscopes. The water in the pasteurization chamber is raised to 75°C and maintained for 10 minutes.

Lifting forceps may be boiled for 10 minutes and the blades placed in a container of Hibitane 5 per cent in 70 per cent spirit.

Requirements for Unsterile Treatments and Investigations

RECORDING TEMPERATURE, PULSE AND RESPIRATION

Clinical thermometers (each patient should have his own thermometer)
Medi-swabs
Rectal thermometers
Lubricant
Medical wipes
Paper bag for soiled swabs
A watch with a second hand
Charts (Temperature)
Red and blue pens

BATHING IN BED

Bath blankets
Hot and cold water
Bucket
Washing bowl
Soap
Face and back flannel
Bath and hand towel
Nail scissors or nail file
Deodorant
Talcum powder
Toothbrush and paste
Brush and comb
Glass of mouthwash

Unsterile Treatments and Investigations

Bowl
Clean gown or pyjamas
Clean bed linen
Dirty linen container
Razor for a man
Screens

BATHING A BABY

Screens
Baby bath
Water at 39°C
Bath thermometer
Low chair
Face mask
Nurse's gown
Mackintosh or plastic apron
Flannel or towelling apron
Bath towel
Rectal thermometer tray
Small bowl of sterile water (warm)
Wool swabs
Receiver or paper bag
Soap
Sponge or flannel
Baby powder
Ung. zinc and castor oil
Fine nail scissors
Safety pins
Hair brush
Clean napkins, clean clothes
Clean cot linen
Dirty linen rounder
Two pails with lids for soiled napkins and clothes
Cord dressings if required
Plastic pants or disposable Paddi pants

MEDICATED BATHS

Savlon concentrate 25 ml ⎫
Ung. Emulsificious 50 g   ⎬ to a bath of water
Liquor picis carb 80–100 ml ⎭

A normal bath holds approximately 115 litre of water

HOT AND COLD BATHS

Temperature of baths
Hot   37°–40.5°C — 98°–105°F
Warm   34°–37°C   — 93°–98°F
Tepid 27°–34°C   — 80°–93°F
Cool   18°–27°C   — 65°–80°F
Cold   13°–18°C   — 55°–65°F

CARE OF THE INCONTINENT PATIENT

Cotton wool or Inco tissues	Back flannel
Bowl lined with paper bag	Towel
Washing bowl	Talcum powder or prescribed ointment
Hot water	Container for foul linen
Soap	Container for dirty linen

Unsterile Treatments and Investigations

Clean drawsheet and sheets
Clean gown
Incontinent pads or disposable Paddi pants
Clean mackintosh or polythene sheet

MOUTH CARE

Paper towel
Bowl with paper bag
Gallipots
Lotions for cleaning mouth, e.g. soda bicarbonate or glycothymol in water
Mouthwash and bowl
Bowl for dentures
Toothbrush and paste
Vaseline petroleum jelly
Tongue depressor
1 pair small sponge-holding forceps
1 pair dissecting forceps
Gauze squares or dental wipes
Mouth gag for unconscious patient

WASHING HAIR IN BED

Mackintoshes or polythene sheets
2 bath towels
Shoulder cape
Face towel
Large jug of water at 37°C
Small jug for rinsing
Sachet or bottle of shampoo
Scissors
Pail
Clean brush and comb

Hairpins, grips, or
  rollers
Hair dryer

Protection for the floor
Washing bowl

COMBING A VERMINOUS HEAD

A good light is
  essential
Mackintosh or
  polythene sheet
Shoulder cape
Paper bag or bowl
  with a lid

Toothcomb
Patient's comb
Large lint squares
Gallipot
Pipette
Suleo lotion or
  Lethane emulsion

NB: Vinegar in water ā ā (equal parts) for removal of nits

IRRIGATION OF THE EYE

Shoulder cape
Towel
Receiver or Fisher's
  dish
Gauze squares or tetra
  swabs
Jug of lotion at 35°C

Lotion thermometer
Undine
Eye pad
Adhesive strapping or,
Pad
Bandage
Safety pin

Lotions. Normal saline, sterile distilled water

Unsterile Treatments and Investigations

Boracic lotion and distilled water
ā ā equal parts.

All equipment must be perfectly clean.
After operations on the eye, the procedure is carried out with full aseptic precautions.

INSTILLATION OF EYE DROPS

Receiver   Prescription sheet
Pipette   Drops as prescribed
Gauze squares or tetra
  swabs

Today many eye drops are dispensed commercially in disposable plastic drop bottles.
Bottles should be discarded after 7 days and used only for the prescribed patient.

APPLICATION OF EYE OINTMENT

Receiver   Ointment prescribed
Glass rods   Prescription sheet
Gauze squares or tetra swabs

Glass rods must be sterilized after use, a separate one being used for each eye.
Today eye ointments are dispensed in tubes with a long nozzle for easy application.

EXAMINATION OF THE EAR, NOSE, AND THROAT

Treatment lamp and head mirror or,
Head lamp and battery
Auriscope
Aural speculae
Aural dressing forceps
Wooden applicators
Wool carriers
Ear wool
1cm ribbon gauze
Ring probe
Tuning fork
Wax hooks
Ear drops
Nasal speculae
Paper handkerchiefs
Nasal forceps
Post nasal mirror
Spirit lamp
Matches
Tongue depressors
Gauze squares
Laryngeal mirrors
Laryngoscope
Sterile swab sticks
Stuart's medium bottles
Laboratory forms
Bowl for dentures
Mouthwash in glass, bowl
Shoulder cape
Cocaine 10 per cent in throat spray
Cocaine ointment 25 per cent
Silver nitrate sticks
Paper bag or receiver

SYRINGING AN EAR

Shoulder cape
Towel
2 receivers
Aural syringe

Unsterile Treatments and Investigations

Jug lotion at 37°C
Lotion thermometer
Wool swabs
Treatment lamp
Head mirror
Auriscope

Wax hook or ringed probe
Warm olive oil drops
Pipette
Paper bag or receiver
Lotions, tap water or normal saline

OPENING A QUINSY

Shoulder cape
Receiver
Treatment lamp and head mirror
Gloves
Tongue depressors
Gauze squares
Sterile scalpel (No. 15 blade on a Bard Parker handle)
Sterile sinus forceps
Vomit bowl and cloth
Hot saline mouthwash
Sterile swabstick
Laboratory form
Bottle of Stuart's medium

N.B. Cocaine 10 per cent in a throat spray may be used as a local analgesic although this is not desirable.

TO OBTAIN A THROAT SWAB

Treatment lamp and head mirror or torch
Receiver or paper bag
Tongue depressor

Sterile swabsticks   Bottle Stuart's
Laboratory form   medium

N.B. Throat swabs are preferably taken in the early morning before eating.

GASTROSTOMY FEEDS

Mackintosh or polythene sheet
Receiver
Diet cloth
Tray and traycloth
Glass funnel ⎫
Tubing   ⎬ in bowl of water
Glass or plastic conical connection ⎭
Spigot

Gate clip
Prepared feed at 37°C
Food thermometer
50 ml of tap water in a small jug
Medicines and/or drugs
Medicine glass
Prescription sheet
Mouthwash or toothbrush and paste

N.B. The patient may wish to chew desired food, in which case a vomit bowl and cloth is required.

OESOPHAGEAL FEED ORAL ROUTE

Shoulder cape   Diet cloth
Receiver   Tray and traycloth

Unsterile Treatments and Investigations

Glass funnel ⎫
Tubing ⎪
Conical connection ⎬ in bowl
Oesophageal tube of suitable size ⎪ of water
5 or 10 ml syringe ⎭
Blue litmus paper   Spigot
Gallipots   Gate clip
Lubricant
Medical wipes
50 ml water in a small jug
Prepared feed 37°C
Food thermometer
Medicine and/or drugs
Medicine glass
Prescription sheet
Vomit bowl and cloth
Mouthwash
Zinc oxide strapping or Micropore

N.B. A mouth gag and mouth cleaning tray will be required if the patient is unconscious.

NASAL ROUTE

Requirements as for oral route
Wisp of wool in warm water or
paper handkerchiefs for cleaning nostrils
Mouth gag not required.

TEST MEAL

Trolley
Shoulder cape
Ryles tube size 12 ⎫
10 ml syringe   ⎭ in a bowl of water
Spigot
Gallipot
Lubricant
Medical wipes
Zinc oxide strapping or Micropore
Rack of 12 specimen bottles
Label
Test meal or laboratory form
Vomit bowl and cloth
Mouthwash
Watch
Paper handkerchiefs or wisp of wool in warm water to clean nostrils

Pentagastrin Test Meal

Dose 6 micrograms of Pentagastrin per kilo body weight
Tuberculin syringe and a No 25 needle
Gauze to strain aspirate

Alcohol Test Meal

50 ml of 70 per cent alcohol in water
Medicine glass

Unsterile Treatments and Investigations

Gruel Test Meal

Cup, saucer and spoon
500 ml gruel
To make gruel—add 15 g fine oatmeal to a litre of water
Boil and reduce to 500 ml

Histamine phosphate injection may be given subcutaneously
Dose 0.25 mg to 0.5 mg

GASTRIC LAVAGE

Trolley
Mackintosh or
   polythene sheet
Shoulder cape
Receiver
Gallipot
Medical wipes
Lubricant
Funnel
Rubber or polythene tubing
Glass or plastic straight connection
Gastric tube
} in a bowl of water

Unsterile Treatments and Investigations

Large jug water at 37°C
Lotion thermometer
1 litre jug
Bowl with lid for gastric residue
Pail
Vomit bowl and cloth
Bowl for dentures
Specimen bottle
Laboratory form
Mouth gag if the patient is unconscious

Lotions: tap water or normal saline

N.B. If the patient is unconscious the trachea should be intubated with a cuffed tube by an anaesthetist.
A Senorans tube and evacuator can be used instead of tube and funnel.

ADMINISTRATION OF MEDICINES

Drug trolley containing:

Drugs and medicines
Medicine glasses
Oil cups
Conical 5 and 10 ml glass measures
Teaspoons
1 ml pipettes
5 ml plastic spoons
Jug of water
Jug of milk
Straws
Pestle and mortar
Jam
Small tray
Bowl hot water
Glass cloth
Prescription sheets

Unsterile Treatments and Investigations

NEUROLOGICAL EXAMINATION

Ophthalmoscope
Sphygmomanometer
Stethoscope
Patella hammer
Tuning fork
2 point discriminator
Pen torch
Laryngeal mirror
Spirit lamp
Matches
Spatulae
Gauze squares or dental wipes
Substances for testing smell and taste, e.g. salt, sugar, cloves, peppermint
Test tubes for hot and cold water
Pins
Cotton wool
Tape measure
Guttae homatropine 1 per cent
Prescription sheet

ADMINISTRATION OF OXYGEN

Nasal route
Oxygen cylinder and key
Flowmeter
Humidifier
Pressure tubing or polythene tubing
Paper handkerchiefs or
Wisps of wool in warm water
Safety pin
Lanolin
1 pr Wallace nasal oxygen cannulae
By Ventimask, 24 per cent, 28 per cent or 35 per cent oxygen

Run oxygen at 4 litres per minute
Oxygen cylinder and key
Pressure tubing or polythene tubing
Flowmeter
Humidifier

By M.C. mask—as above omitting ventimask
Run oxygen at 2 litres per minute
(M.C.=Mary Cantrell)

OXYGEN TENT

Oxygen cylinder and key
Flowmeter
Humidifier
Oxygen tent
Room thermometer
Safety pin or string
Bowl to drain refrigeration unit

N.B. A long mackintosh or polythene sheet should be placed under the mattress whenever possible.

APPLICATION OF PLASTER

Plaster bandages of various sizes
Stockinette
Adhesive felt
Plaster wool
Bucket of tepid water
Plaster knife
Plaster shears
Plaster benders
Plaster scissors

Unsterile Treatments and Investigations

Mackintoshes or polythene sheets
Mackintosh or polythene apron
Gown
Plaster boots
Dust sheets or newspapers
Tape measure
Skin pencil
Olive oil
Wool swabs
Materials for washing and shaving the skin may be required

REMOVAL OF PLASTER

Mackintosh or polythene apron
Mackintosh or polythene sheet
Dust sheet or newspapers
Plaster shears
Plaster benders
Plaster knife
Electric plaster circular saw
Plaster scissors
Container for plaster
Materials for washing skin
Olive oil and wool swabs
Sterile dressings if required

KAOLIN POULTICE (ANTIPHLOGISTINE)

Poultice board or slab
Spatula in jug of hot water
Container of kaolin
Saucepan of boiling water

White lint	Safety-pins
Gauze	2 warmed receivers or bowls
White wool	
Bandage	Pair of scissors

N.B. There is now a commercially packed poultice backed with aluminium foil. The plastic cover is cut away and the kaolin covered with gauze, then used in the usual manner.

ICE POULTICE

Board or slab	Non-absorbent wool
Ice	Adhesive plaster
Ice pick	Lint
Salt	Bandage } in a
Teaspoon	Safety-pin } receiver
Protective tissue, e.g. oiled silk, jaconet	

ICE BAG

Ice cubes	Bed cradle } may be
Salt	String } required
Teaspoon	
Ice bag with cover or polythene bag	

Unsterile Treatments and Investigations

STARCH POULTICE

Poultice board or slab
Large bowl
Palette knife
Wooden spoon
Tablespoon
Teaspoon
Jug of cold water

Kettle of boiling water
Starch
Boracic powder
Old linen
Bandage
Safety-pins
Receiver or paper bag

RECTAL EXAMINATION

Tray
Incontinence pad
Disposable gloves
Finger stalls with cape

Medical wipes
Rectal lubricant
Proctoscope
Light

Position: left lateral

SIGMOIDOSCOPY

Trolley
Sigmoidoscope
Light carrier
2 wool carriers
Biopsy forceps
Receiver

Wool swabs
Gauze squares
Rectal lubricant
Finger stalls with cape
  or
Rubber gloves

Unsterile Treatments and Investigations

Proctoscope and light
Battery
Bellows
Light lead
Specimen bottle
  containing
  Formal-saline
Laboratory form
Plastic apron or gown
Mackintosh or
  polythene sheet

Position: left lateral or knee chest

PURGATIVE ENEMA

Incontinence pad
Tray
Receiver
Rectal tube ⎫
Funnel   ⎬ size 14
Tubing   ⎬ French
Connection ⎬ gauge
Gate clip   ⎭
Lubricant
Medical wipes
Jug
Lotion thermometer
Bed pan or commode
Toilet roll

or
Disposable phosphate enema

Solutions: Tap water 500 millilitre at 37°C
           Soft soap 25 millilitre to 475 millilitre
             of water
           Glycerine 8–16 millilitre to 30 millilitre
             of water
Position: left lateral

Unsterile Treatments and Investigations

RECTAL LAVAGE

Incontinence pad
Receiver
Rectal lubricant
Medical wipes
Rectal tube size 14 French gauge or Charrière gauge
Tubing
Connection

Funnel
Large jug of water at 37°C
1 litre jug
Lotion thermometer
Pail
Bed pan or commode } may be required
Toilet roll

Position: left lateral

COLONIC LAVAGE

As for rectal lavage
Bed elevator or bed blocks

PASSING A FLATUS TUBE

Incontinence pad
Bowl of disinfectant, e.g. carbolic lotion 5 per cent

Flatus tube size 16
Medical wipes
Rectal lubricant
Bowl or paper bag

Position: left lateral

SHAVING

- Mackintosh or polythene sheet
- Tray
- Razor and blades
- Bowl of hot water
- Towel
- Wool swabs
- Washing bowl
- Soap and flannel
- Talcum powder
- Bowl or paper bag

N.B. A good light is necessary.

SKIN TRACTION

- Mackintosh or polythene sheet
- Materials for washing and shaving the skin
- Extension Elastoplast
- Spreader or stirrup
- Cord
- Weights
- Pulleys
- Cotton and crêpe bandages
- Pad of wool or sorbo
- Adhesive felt
- Scissors
- Tape measure
- Bed elevator
- Balkan beam or Hoskin's frame
- Hamilton-Russell sling
- Pillow } or
- Thomas splint
- Flannel strips
- Safety-pins
- Tincture of benzoin compound in spray bottle

Unsterile Treatments and Investigations

STEAM INHALATION

Mackintosh or polythene sheet
Shoulder cape
Nelson inhaler with a glass mouthpiece
Gauze square
Inhaler cover or towel
Boiling water
Cold water
Jug
Measure
Medication; e.g. tincture benzoin compound
Sputum carton or paper handkerchiefs
Pillow covered with a waterproof case

TEPID SPONGING

Thermometer tray
Temperature chart
Bath thermometer
Washing bowl
Jug of water at 32°C reduce to 21°C
Bowl of ice
2 to 6 sponges
Face towel
Compresses in iced water
Cool drink
Electric fan
Bed cradle
Clean bed linen
Clean cotton gown
Soiled linen container

N.B. Reduce temperature of patient by not more than 2°C.

VAGINAL DOUCHE

Mackintosh or
  polythene sheet
Douche can
Rubber tubing
Glass douche nozzle,
  gate clip or,
Connection }
Jacques catheter }
Wool swabs

Bowl of antiseptic
  solution at 37°C
Lotion thermometer
Bedpan and cover
Treatment lamp
Sanitary pad and belt
Talcum powder

Lotions: normal saline, lactic acid 1 per cent,
         soda bicarbonate 1.7 g to 500 ml water

HIGH VAGINAL SWAB

Mackintosh or
  polythene sheet
Treatment lamp
Wool swabs
Bowl of normal saline } sterile
Sims' or Cusco's
  vaginal speculum
Sterile swabstick
Bottle Stuart's
  medium
Laboratory form

Unsterile Treatments and Investigations

CERVICAL SMEAR (PAPANICALOU SMEAR)

Mackintosh or polythene sheet
Sims' vaginal speculum
Ayers spatula
Glass slides
Plastic holder containing preservative solution
Investigation form
Pen or pencil

VAGINAL EXAMINATION

Mackintosh or polythene sheet
2 receivers
Anglepoise lamp
Rubber gloves, various sizes
Disposable polythene gloves (all sizes)
Glove powder
Lubricant
Wool swabs
Sanitary pads
Sterile swabsticks
Equipment for taking cervical smears
Laboratory forms
Sims' vaginal speculae (large, medium and small)
Cusco's vaginal speculae (large, medium and small)
Long sponge holding forceps
Vulsellum forceps
Playfair's probe
Rectal tray
Normal saline
Paper bags for soiled equipment

INSERTION OF PESSARIES

Requirements for a vaginal douche
Hodge's pessaries of various sizes
P.V.C. ring pessaries of various sizes
Rubber gloves
Glove powder
Sims' vaginal speculum

Requirements for Aseptic Techniques

The requirements for many of the following procedures are the same and so the details of the Basic Trolley will not be repeated every time.

Basic trolley

Sterile pack containing
- 2 gallipots
- 2 pairs dressing forceps
- Dressing towels
- Gauze squares
- Wool swabs

2 ml syringe
Hypodermic needles } sterile
Lifting forceps

Skin cleaning lotion
Local analgesic e.g. lignocaine ½ or 1 per cent
Mackintosh or polythene sheet

ACUPUNCTURE

Dressing trolley
Extra sterile cotton towels
Soap and flannel
Towel
Masks

Sterile Bard Parker handle with a number 15 blade
Washing bowl
Cotton bandages
Mackintoshes or polythene sheets
A tray for shaving may be required

ANTRUM PUNCTURE AND WASHOUT

Shoulder cape
Receiver for soiled instruments
Lamp and head mirror
Cocaine ointment 25 per cent
Lotion thermometer
Lifting forceps (sterile)
2 specimen bottles
Laboratory form
Bowl 14 cm
Paper handkerchiefs
Mouthwash
2 nasal speculae ⎫
2 Lichtwitz' trocar and cannulae ⎪
Antral syringe or Higginson's syringe ⎬ sterile
Jug containing normal saline 37°C ⎭
Cotton wool balls
Wooden applicators

FEMALE CATHETERIZATION

A good light is essential
Mackintosh or polythene sheet
Receiver for soiled swabs
Lifting forceps
Measuring jug
Specimen bottle
Laboratory form

Requirements for Aseptic Techniques

Warm antiseptic
  solution
Sterile lubricant e.g.
  K.Y. Jelly

Dressing towel ⎫
Wool swabs ⎪
Bowl ⎪
Gauze squares to
  apply lubricant to
  catheters ⎬ sterile
2 Jacques catheters
  size 6 French gauge ⎪
2 dressing forceps ⎪
Receiver ⎭

Position: dorsal with knees flexed and abducted

See Foley catheter page 27 for continuous bladder drainage.

MALE CATHETERIZATION

A good light is essential
Mackintosh or polythene sheets
Receiver for soiled swabs
Measuring jug
Specimen bottle
Laboratory form
Tube of analgesic lubricant e.g. Xylotox Gel.
Warm antiseptic lotion

- Dressing towels
- Bowl
- Wool swabs
- Gauze squares
- 2 pair dressing forceps
- Catheters, several sizes and types of rubber and gum elastic
- Catheter introducer
- Nozzle for lubricant
- Receiver

} sterile

For use with a Foley catheter (continuous bladder drainage)

- 10 ml syringe
- Water
- Catheter drainage bag

} sterile

- Drainage bag stand
- Gate clip
- Adhesive strapping
- Safety pin

Requirements for Aseptic Techniques

BLADDER LAVAGE

Catheter in situ
Receiver
Bladder syringe
or
Funnel ⎫
Tubing ⎪
Connection ⎬
Gate clip ⎭
Measuring jug ⎬ sterile
Lotion at 37°C
Large bowl or pail
Mackintosh or
 polythene sheet
Lotion thermometer

Lotions: sterile distilled water or sterile normal saline.

CLEAN SPECIMEN OF URINE—FEMALE

Bowl of warm
 antiseptic lotion ⎫
Wool swabs ⎬ sterile
Measuring jug ⎭
Specimen bottle

Laboratory form
Bed pan and cover
Soap and flannel ⎱ may be used instead of anti-
Towel ⎰ septic lotion and wool swabs

MID STREAM SPECIMEN OF URINE—MALE

Bowl of warm
   antiseptic solution
Wool swabs   ⎬ sterile
Measuring jug
Funnel
Specimen bottle
Laboratory form
Urinal

INTRAMUSCULAR AND HYPODERMIC INJECTIONS

Tray
Medi-swabs
Sterile syringes 1, 2
   and 5 ml

Selection of sterile
   needles
Drug prescribed
Prescription sheet

N.B. Not more than 4 ml should be injected into one site.

Requirements for Aseptic Techniques

Injection of Serum

As for intramuscular injection with the addition of:

Adrenaline 1–1,000	1 ml syringe and subcutaneous needles
Antihistamine drug, e.g. Piriton	
Hydrocortisone	

N.B. Oxygen should be readily available.

INTRAVENOUS PENTOTHAL

- Receiver
- Medi-swabs
- Sterile 20 ml syringe with an eccentric nozzle
- Size 1 hypodermic needle
- Ampoules of sodium pentothal 1 g
- Sterile distilled water
- Pentothal mixer
- Tourniquet
- 2 sterile hypodermic syringes and needles
- Adrenaline 1–1,000, Megimide, Hydrocortisone and nikethamide
- Oxygen equipment
- Mouth gag
- Tongue forceps
- Sponge holding forceps
- Gauze squares or dental wipes
- Airways and lubricant
- Vomit bowl and cloth
- Pulse chart
- Anaesthetic consent form

INTRAVENOUS INFUSION OR BLOOD TRANSFUSION

Basic trolley
Butterfly cannulae

- 0.6 mm or size 23
- 0.8 mm or size 21
- 1.1 mm or size 19

sterile
mm = millimetre

Venflon cannulae
Sterile intravenous giving set
Sphygmomanometer
or
Tourniquet
Intravenous stand
Splint
Bandage and safety pin
Adhesive strapping
Pillow with protective cover
Vacolitre of normal saline, glucose 5 per cent, blood or other solution for infusion
Temperature, pulse and respiration chart if blood is given.

Requirements for Aseptic Techniques

It may be necessary to cut down onto a vein, therefore the following equipment should be available.

- Scalpel
- 2 pairs fine toothed dissecting forceps
- 2 pairs small artery forceps
- 1 pair small scissors
- 1 aneurysm needle
- Small curved cutting needle
- Fine plain catgut
- Nylon sutures
- Face masks
- Rubber gloves

} sterile

CENTRAL VENOUS PRESSURE LINE

Basic trolley
Bard Parker handle Number 15 blade
Bard–I–Cath 12" intravenous catheter
Intravenous giving set
Intravenous stand
Central venous pressure manometer set
Manometer
Fluid balance chart
Central venous pressure chart

N.B. The venous pressure is read as millimetre of water.

The jugular vein is the most common vein used.

TAKING BLOOD FROM A DONOR

Basic trolley
Blood taking set
Blood collecting bottle containing 125 ml acid citrate dextrose
or
Blood collecting bag containing 75 ml acid citrate dextrose
Sphygmomanometer or tourniquet
Blood bottles, bags and taking sets are usually obtained from the local Blood Transfusion centre.
Cross matching bottle.

N.B. After giving blood the donor should rest for half an hour, and should be given a cup of tea and biscuits.

BLOOD CULTURE

1 10 ml syringe
2 No 1 needles
Medi-swabs
Three blood culture bottles
A and B contain Castenda's medium (penicillinase)
Bottle C contains Robertson's meat broth
Laboratory form
Sphygmomanometer or tourniquet
Receiver for soiled swabs

Requirements for Aseptic Techniques

BLOOD GROUPING

INTERNATIONAL CLASSIFICATION
Provided the Rhesus factor is compatible:
Group A can receive from Group A.O.
Group B can receive from Group B.O.
Group AB. Universal recipient.
Group O. Universal donor, can only receive from Group O.

SUBCUTANEOUS INFUSION

Basic trolley
Intravenous giving set
Vacolitre of normal saline or Hartmann's solution
No. 1 hypodermic needle
2 ml hypodermic syringe
Ampoule hyalase 1,500 international units
Ampoule sterile water 2 ml
Adhesive strapping
Fluid balance chart
Intravenous stand

SIMPLE DRESSING

Mackintosh or polythene sheet if necessary
Container for soiled dressings

Container for soiled instruments
Lifting forceps
Adhesive strapping, Micropore or Elastoplast

2 gallipots
2 receivers
4 pairs dressing forceps } sterile
Dressing towel
Dressings

Bandages
Safety pins
Face masks if required
Skin cleaning lotions
Hand towel

Removal of sutures

As for simple dressing. In addition stitch scissors or stitch cutter

Removal of clips

As for simple dressing
1 pair Michel clip removers or a pair of artery forceps for butterfly clips

Surgical preparation of the skin

As for simple dressing

Extra cotton sterile towels

Materials for washing and shaving the skin
Cotton bandages

Requirements for Aseptic Techniques

SUTURING A WOUND

A basic trolley
Scissors
1 pair toothed dissecting forceps
Needle holder
Curved cutting needles
Nylon suture
Scalpel ⎫
Probe ⎪
Sinus forceps ⎪
2 pairs artery forceps ⎬ these may be required
Rubber and gauze ⎪ for other than clean
  drains ⎪ stitched wounds
Safety pins ⎪
Catgut ⎪
Rubber gloves ⎭

N.B. An anaesthetic may be given, in which case a consent form will be required.

OPENING AN ABSCESS

As for a simple dressing.
In addition:
1 sinus forceps ⎫
1 silver probe ⎬ sterile
1 Volkmann's spoon ⎭
Scalpel

1 pair of scissors ⎫
Rubber and gauze
  drains   ⎬ sterile
Safety-pins
Rubber gloves ⎭
Gown and mask   Local analgesia may
Swabstick   be given but more
Stuart's medium   often a general
Laboratory form   anaesthetic
                            Consent form

LUMBAR PUNCTURE

Basic trolley   Laboratory form
2 sterile lumbar   2 per cent liq. iodine
  puncture needles   Adhesive dressing or
Sterile manometer,   collodion flex
  tubing and   Face masks and gloves
  connection   Bed elevator or blocks
2 specimen bottles   may be required

Position: the patient should be lying on a firm surface in the left lateral position, with the knees drawn up under the chin.

PARACENTESIS ABDOMINIS
(Tapping the Abdomen)

Basic trolley

Requirements for Aseptic Techniques

Scalpel	
Robert's trocar and cannula	
2 lengths of tubing	} sterile
Glass drip connection	
Drainage bag	
Many-tailed bandage	Face masks
Safety-pins	Gloves
Adhesive strapping	Specimen bottle
Gate clip	Laboratory form
	Fluid chart

N.B. The patient must empty his bladder. Catheterization may be necessary.

PERITONEAL DIALYSIS

Basic trolley		Peritoneal dialysis drainage bag
Lifting forceps		
Bard Parker handle and a No 11 blade		Curved cutting needle
Hypodermic needles No's 1 and 25	} sterile {	Needle holder
Peritoneal dialysis catheter. 'Trocath' 12 inches		Nylon suture
		Scissors
		Gloves
Y type peritoneal giving set		3 extra cotton towels

Intravenous stand
Containers of dialysate
  1.36 per cent dextrose
  6.36 per cent
    dextrose*
  Dialysis sheet
Heparin
Potassium
2 ml syringe

No. 1 needle
Label for additives
  to dialysate
Masks
Elastoplast
Warming chamber
  for dialysate
Bed cradle

A L.K.B. Medical AB dialyser can be used instead of the containers of dialysate

* This solution is only used when the patient is oedematous or over dialised.

N.B. If not anuric the patient must empty his bladder.

PARACENTESIS THORACIS
(Chest Aspiration)

Basic trolley
50 ml syringe
Chest aspirating needles of various lengths and size ⎫
Two-way tap ⎬ sterile
Rubber tubing and sinker ⎭
Measuring jug

Requirements for Aseptic Techniques

Specimen bottle
Laboratory form
Sputum cup or paper handkerchiefs
Sedative cough medicine, e.g. linctus codeine
Medicine glass
Prescription sheet
Adhesive dressing or collodion flex
Face masks
Gloves

Position: sitting up leaning forward over a bed-table or supported in the lateral position. Patient's X-rays should be available.

ASPIRATION OF A PNEUMOTHORAX

Basic trolley
2 sterile pneumothorax needles and rubber tubing
Maxwell box
Masks and gloves
Sedative cough linctus e.g. linctus codeine
Prescription sheet

Position: either lateral, exposing affected side, a pillow under the chest and the arm extended above the head;
or leaning forward over a bed table.

A thoracotomy drain and under water seal drainage bottle may be used for this procedure, in which case a Robert's suction apparatus will be required.

TRACHEOTOMY

Basic trolley

sterile:
- 1 scalpel
- 4 pairs artery forceps
- 2 pairs toothed dissecting forceps
- 1 pair scissors
- 2 double hooked retractors
- 1 blunt hook
- 1 sharp hook
- Tracheal dilators
- Tracheotomy tubes of various types and size
- Suction catheters
- Curved cutting needles
- Nylon skin sutures
- Fine plain catgut
- Needle holder
- Rubber gloves and glove powder

Suction apparatus
Face masks
Tulle Gras or vaseline gauze
Sandbag
Tape for tracheotomy tubes

A very good light

Requirements for Aseptic Techniques

CARE OF TRACHEOTOMY

- Mackintosh or polythene sheet
- Bowl of soda bicarbonate solution
- Tracheotomy tube brush or pipe cleaners
- Face masks
- Tulle Gras or vaseline gauze
- Paper handkerchiefs
- Suction apparatus
- Bowl of sterile water for cleaning catheters after use with suction

Sterile:
- Dressings
- Suction catheters
- Spare tracheotomy tubes the same size as the one in situ
- Tracheal dilators
- 2 pairs dressing forceps

Disposable polythene gloves

N.B. Writing paper, pencil, mirror and bell will be required by the patient.

Weights and Measures

APOTHECARIES CAPACITY MEASURE

60 minims	= 1 drachm
8 fluid drachms	= 1 fluid ounce
20 ounces	= 1 pint
2 pints	= 1 quart
4 quarts	= 1 gallon

Not now in common use.

METRIC MEASURES IN S.I. UNITS

S.I. units = Système International d'Unités or International System of Units

Common Symbols and conversion factors

Weight μg = microgram = 1 000 000 of a gram
mg = milligram = 1 000 ,, ,,
g = gram = 1·0
kg = kilogram = 1 000·0 gram

Weights and Measures

```
1 g  =   0·035 of an ounce
1 kg =   2·2   pounds
1 oz =  28·35  gram
1 lb = 453·6   gram
1 st =   6·35  kilogram
```

1 microgram	=	0·000 001	gram
1 milligram	=	0·001	,,
1 centigram	=	0·01	,,
1 gram	=	1·0	
1 decagram	=	10·0	gram
1 hectogram	=	100·0	,,
1 kilogram	= 1	000·0	,,

MOLECULAR UNITS

Mol = mole—for molecular substances, this is the molecular weight in grammes

mmol	= millimole	= 0·001	of a mole
μ mol	= micromole	= 0·000 001	,, ,,
n mol	= nanomole	= 0·000 000 001	,, ,,

VOLUME

ml	= millilitre	= 0·001 of a litre
cl	= centilitre	= 0·01 ,, ,,

dl	= decilitre	= 0·1 of a litre
L	= litre	= 1·0 litre

1 fluid ounce = 28·4 ml
1 pint = 568·0 ml

LENGTH

μm	= micrometre	= 0·000001 of a metre		
mm	= millimetre	= 0·001	,,	,,
cm	= centimetre	= 0·01	,,	,,
m	= metre	= 1·0	,,	,,

25·4 mm = 1 inch
2·54 cm = 1 inch
0·30 m = 1 foot
0·91 m = 1 yard

The symbol S should not be added to make plurals. In S.I. units S = seconds.

PRESSURE

The unit of pressure is a pascal. **These units are not yet in general use.**

μPa	= micropascal	= 0·000 001 of a pascal
mPa	= millipascal	= 0·001

Weights and Measures

kPa	= kilopascal	= 1·0 pascal
MPa	= megapascal	= 1 000 000 pascal
GPa	= gigapascal	= 1 000 000 000 pascal

This unit should be used in place of measuring mm Hg in measuring blood pressure

1 mm Hg = 133·3 Pa   150 mm Hg = 20 kilopascal

Hg = mercury

TIME

24 hour clock

   1 AM–12 MD as usual
   1 PM–12 MN = 13.00 hrs–24.00 hrs

THERMOMETRIC EQUIVALENTS

Celsius		Fahrenheit
35·0°	=	95·0°
36·2°	=	97·2°
36·8°	=	98·2°
37·8°	=	100·0°
38·4°	=	101·0°
39·0°	=	102·2°

39·8°	=	103·6°
40·2°	=	104·4°
41·0°	=	105·8°

To convert °F to °C subtract 32, multiply by $\frac{5}{9}$
e.g. 101°F − 32 = 69 × $\frac{5}{9}$ = 38·3°C

To convert °C to °F multiply by $\frac{9}{5}$ and then add 32
e.g. 37°C × $\frac{9}{5}$ = 66·6 + 32 = 98·6°F

Dilution of Lotions

Example 1

Make 500 ml of carbolic lotion 1 in 80 from a 1 in 20 solution.
Required solution is a $\frac{1}{4}$ strength of the given solution.
Therefore divide 1 in 20 by 1 in 80 $1/80 \times 20/1 = \frac{1}{4}$
$\frac{1}{4}$ of 500 ml is 125 ml of carbolic lotion
1 in 20 and 375 ml of water to give the strength of the carbolic lotion required.

Example 2

To make 500 ml of Hibitane 1 in 5,000 from a 1 in 1,000 solution.
Required solution is 1/5 strength of given solution.
Divide 1 in 1,000 by 1 in 5,000 $1/5000 \times 1/1000 = 1/5$ of 500 ml.
One fifth of 500 ml = 100 ml of Hibitane 1 in 1,000 and 400 ml of water.

Example 3

To make 250 ml of a 1 per cent solution of carbolic lotion from a 1 in 20 solution.
One per cent solution is 1 in 100
Divide 1 in 20 by 1 in 100 $1/100 \times 20/1 = 1/5$
One fifth of 250 ml is 50 ml
∴ 50 ml of carbolic 1 in 20
   200 ml of water is required.

Pharmacy Act 1971

The Misuse of Drugs Act came into existence in 1971 (Controlled Drugs Act)

Regulations made under this act restrict the use of habit forming drugs. Included are:

Amphetamine	
Benzphetamine	(Didrex)
Chlorphentermine	(Lucefen)
Cocaine	
Dexamphetamine	
Dextromoramide	(Palfium)
Diamorphine	
Diconal	
Dihydrocodeine injection	(D.F.118)
Fentanyl	
Hydromorphone	(Dilaudid)
Leverphanol	(Dromoran)
Mephenternine	(Mephine)
Methadone	
Methaqualone	(in Mandrax)

Methylamphetamine
Methylphenidate (Ritalin)
Morphine
Papaveretum (Omnopon)
Pethidine
Phenazocine (Narphen)
Phenmetrazin (Preludin)
Phenoperidine

Poisons and Pharmacy Act 1933

This act is to be repealed in the near future and will be known as The Poisons Act 1972.
The poison rules made under this act control the supply and sale of poisonous substances.
Among the drugs included in the various Schedule of Rules are:

Acetanilide
Alkaloids and their salts including:

Atropine
Codeine
Colchicine
Curare
Emetine
Ephedrine
Ergometrine
Ergotamine
Hyoscine
Hyoscyamine
Lobelia
Strychnine

Amidopyrine
Antihistamines
Barbituric Acid its salts and derivatives
Digitalis glycosides
Dihydrocodeine DF118 ORAL
Insulin

Sulphonamides
Thyroid
Most of the tranquillizers and anti-depressants.

Many of the drugs included are available on prescription only. The preparation and supply of antibiotics, corticosteroids, and other biological preparations are controlled by the Therapeutic Substances Act 1956 (again shortly to be repealed).

Latin Abbreviations

a.c.	ante cibos	before meals
ad. lib.	ad libitum	to the desired amount
ā ā	ana	of each
alt. hor.	alternis horis	alternate hours
aq. dest.	aqua destillata	distilled water
b.d.	bis die	twice a day
b.i.d.	bis in die	twice a day
cat.	cataplasma	a poultice
c.c.	cum cibis	with food
c.m.	cras mane	tomorrow morning
c.n.	cras nocte	tomorrow night
comp.	compositus	compounded of
dieb. alt.	diebus alternis	on alternate days
emp.	emplastrum	a plaster
ext.	extractum	extract
gutt.	gutta or guttae	drop or drops
h.n.	hac nocte	tonight
h.s.	hora somni	at bedtime
inf.	infusum	an infusion
inj.	injectio	an injection

o.h.	omni hora	every hour
o.m.	omni mane	every morning
o.n.	omni nocte	every night
part. aeq.	partes aequale	equal parts
p.r.	per rectum	by the rectum
p.r.n.	pro re nata	as occasion arise
pulv.	pulvis	powder
p.v.	per vaginam	by the vagina
q.d.	quater in die	four times a day
q.h.	quater horis	four hourly
q.l.	quantum libet	as much as is wanted
℞	recipe	take
rep.	repetatur	let it be repeated
rep. sem.	repetatur semel	let it be repeated once only
s.s.	semis	a half
sig.	signatur	let it be labelled
stat.	statim	immediately
t.d.s.	ter in die sumendum	let it be taken three times a day
ung.	unguentum	ointment

Food Values

Unit   1 kilocalorie   unit of energy

The Calorie or kilocalorie used in nutrition is the amount of heat required to raise the temperature of 1,000 gram of water 1 degree Celsius, e.g. 15°C to 16°C.

The word calorie used in nutrition should be written with a capital C.

Energy value   Unit   1 Joule   Metric

The unit of energy is the kilojoule. It is the amount of energy expended when 1 kilogram is moved 1 metre by a force of 1 Newton.

A Newton is the force applied to a mass of 1 kilogram, gives it an acceleration of 1 metre per second squared.

Food Values

ENERGY YIELD

1 gram protein	= 4·1 kilocalorie
	= 17·1544 kilojoule
1 gram carbohydrate	= 3·75 kilocalorie
	15·69 kilojoule
1 gram fat	= 9·3 kilocalorie
	38·9112 kilojoule

1 kilocalorie = 4·184 kilojoule. To convert 1 kilocalorie to kilojoule multiply the number of Calories by 4·184

1 000 joule = 1 kilojoule
1 000 000 joule = 1 megajoule

DAILY ENERGY REQUIREMENTS

Average man	3,000 kcal or 12·6 megajoule
Average woman	2,200 kcal or 9·2 megajoule
Pregnant woman	2,400 kcal or 10·0 megajoule
Nursing mother	2,700 kcal or 11·0 megajoule
Boy aged 12 to 15 years	2,800 kcal or 11·7 megajoule
Girl aged 12 to 15 years	2,300 kcal or 9·6 megajoule
Boy aged 15 to 18 years	3,000 kcal or 12·6 megajoule
Girl aged 15 to 18 years	2,300 kcal or 9·6 megajoule
Patient in bed	1,800 to 2,000 or 7·35 to 8·40
Baby	110 kcal to 120 kcal per kilo of body weight = 4·60 kjoule to 5·02 kjoule per kilo of body weight

Food Values

ENERGY VALUES OF SOME FOODS

Composition per ounce or 28.35 gramme

Cow's milk	18 kcalorie or	77 kjoule
Sugar	112 kcalorie or	469 kjoule
Single cream	54 kcalorie or	225 kjoule
White bread	253 kcalorie or	1,060 kjoule
Butter	211 kcalorie or	884 kjoule
Average egg	45 kcalorie or	188 kjoule
Cheddar cheese	117 kcalorie or	490 kjoule
Cottage cheese	32 kcalorie or	137 kjoule
Cooked lean beef	89 kcalorie or	373 kjoule
Cooked chicken	52 kcalorie or	219 kjoule
White fish	19 kcalorie or	82 kjoule
Potato boiled	23 kcalorie or	94 kjoule

Some foods rich in:

Protein meat, fish, eggs, cheese, soya beans and nuts, milk.

Carbohydrate sugar, cereals, potatoes, bread, flour and dried fruits.

Fat Butter, cream, cheese, eggs, and vegetable oils.

Calcium	cheese, egg yolk, milk, carrots, cabbage, ice cream.
Phosphorus	cheese, egg yolk, mackerel, halibut, cod, and liver.
Potassium	prunes, potatoes (raw), sprouts, liver, milk, eggs, cheddar cheese, bacon.
Iron	liver, kidney, eggs, beef, cocoa, wholemeal bread, and dried apricots.
Vitamin A	carrots, halibut liver oil, cod liver oil, liver, butter, cheese, eggs and milk.
Vitamin B	yeast, Marmite, Bemax, wholemeal bread, peanuts and egg yolk.
Vitamin C	Citrous fruits, watercress, sprouts and cabbage.
Vitamin D	cod liver oil, halibut liver oil, herrings, milk, cheese, butter, milk and eggs.

Food Values

Vitamin E   wheat germ, meat and eggs.

Vitamin K   liver.

Urine Testing

Routine Examination

Note colour, smell, amount and naked eye deposits.
A brick-red deposit denotes the presence of urates.
A white cloudy deposit denotes the presence of phosphates or protein.

The Reaction

Dip a strip of litmus paper into the urine.
Blue litmus paper turns red when the urine is acid.
Red litmus paper turns blue when the urine is alkaline.

Specific Gravity

Place the urine in a deep enough glass to allow the urinometer to float. Stand the specimen glass on an even surface and take a reading at eye-level.
Normal specific gravity 1010–1015.

URINE TESTING WITH BILI-LABSTIX

Test for pH, protein, glucose, ketones, bilirubin and blood in the urine.

General Information

1) Bili-Labstix should be stored at a temperature of under 36°C.
2) Do not store in a refrigerator.
3) Avoid exposing to moisture, direct sunlight, heat, acid, alkali or volatile fumes.
4) Do not touch the test areas of the reagent strip.
5) Keep reagent strip away from detergents which may be found in specimen containers and on working surfaces.
6) Do not remove desiccant from bottle.
7) Replace cap of bottle immediately and tightly after removing reagent strip.
8) Read result carefully at the time specified in a good light with the test area held near the colour chart on the bottle label.
9) Do not transfer reagent strips to another bottle.
10) **Do not use strip if any test area is discoloured.**

The specimen of urine

Use a freshly voided unchilled specimen only. A stale specimen gives a false reaction to some of the tests.

DIRECTIONS FOR USE

Completely immerse all reagent areas of the strip in fresh well mixed uncentrifuged urine and remove immediately. Tap the reagent stick on the edge of the urine container to remove excess urine. Compare test areas closely with the corresponding colour charts on the bottle at the time specified. Hold strip close to colour blocks and match quickly. If this instruction is not carried out carefully, faint colour development in the bilirubin reagent area may be overlooked and the test result reported as negative although bilirubin is present. If the test is negative but the presence of bilirubin is suspected retest the specimen with Ictotest reagent tablets.

INTERPRETATIONS OF COLOUR REACTIONS

The user must bear in mind that test results with Bili-labstix are indicative rather than definite or quantitive.

pH

pH values may be interpolated to one-half unit within a range of 5–9.

Urine Testing

Protein

A colour matching any block marked with a + sign indicates significant proteinuria.

Glucose

Light generally indicates 0.25 g per 100 ml of urine or less.
Dark indicates 0.5 g per 100 ml of urine.
Medium indicates glucose is present but does not denote amount.

Ketones

The shade of lavender or purple developed in 15 seconds indicates a small, moderate or large concentration of ketones in the specimen.

Bilirubin

The shades of brown developed at 20 seconds are read as small +, moderate ++ or large +++.

Blood

The shade of blue developed after 30 seconds indicates a small, moderate or large urinary concentration of blood (R.B. Cells or Haemoglobin).

For quantitative tests a 24 hour specimen of urine is sent to the laboratory where a random specimen is taken and analysed.
Millistix has the added reagent for testing the presence of urobilinogen in the urine.

Quantative test for albumen

Take a freshly voided specimen of urine.
Test the reaction, if alkaline, add a few drops of acetic acid. Stir well.
Fill an Esbach's albuminometer up to the letter U with urine. Add Esbach's reagent up to the letter R. Invert the tube and allow the fluids to mix. Stand upright, label and read after 24 hours.
A sediment is shown as parts of albumin per 1,000 or if divided by 10 the percentage.
If the specific gravity of the urine is greater than 1020, dilute the urine with an equal quantity of water. Record the dilution on the label. Multiply the result by two.

Special Tests

ESTIMATION OF BLOOD PRESSURE

Make the patient comfortable. Lift up the sleeve to clear the upper arm without it getting too tight. Abduct the arm a little way from the chest, and see that it is supported and relaxed.

Place the sphygmomanometer in a position where the mercury can easily be seen. The gauge must be vertical. Apply the cuff above the elbow and attach to the mercury gauge. With one hand pump up the cuff and with the other feel the patient's pulse at the wrist, continue to pump until the pulse disappears.

By means of the valve allow the air to escape very gradually so that the pressure falls, watching the manometer but concentrating upon the return of the pulse at the wrist. Immediately the pulse returns, read the gauge, this will give the systolic pressure in millimetres of mercury.

For accurate estimation of both systolic and diastolic pressure repeat as before until the cuff is inflated. A stethoscope is placed on the brachial artery just below the cuff. Open the valve so that compression is gradually reduced until the tapping sounds produced by the pulse wave are heard. Immediately take a reading. This is the systolic pressure. Continue to listen whilst the mercury falls, the sounds persist, but often change in character. Ignore these changes until they become soft and almost inaudible. Take the reading at this point also. This is the diastolic pressure.

Normal systolic pressure is approximately 100 to 140 mm Hg, and the normal diastolic 60 to 90 mm Hg. (mm Hg = millimetres of mercury).

COLONOSCOPY

A colonoscope consists of a firm flexible plastic tube with a controllable end bearing a light and sometimes a camera lens, with which the entire colon can be examined. Vision is made possible by fibro-optics as in the flexible gastroscope but the colonoscope is much longer and the glass fibres are more easily damaged by bending.

This means that only a limited number of colonoscopes can be carried out before the instrument requires costly repair.

Special Tests

Preparation of the Patient

This involves a 3 day regime.

1. From day 1 the patient is given a low-residue diet.
2. On day 2 at 3 pm castor oil 30 millilitre is given by mouth. In the evening a 5 litre tap water enema is administered.

No further food is permitted, but the patient may drink surgical fluids, e.g. clear fluids.

3. On the day of colonoscopy a further 5 litre tap water enema is given 1 hour before the examination is to take place.
4. Valium 10 milligram is given intravenously prior to the examination.
5. The colonoscopy is usually performed in a special room with a table on which the patient lies in the left lateral position.
6. The colonoscope is passed through the anus and its progress is monitored by X-ray.

It may cause psychological and physical discomfort and the nurse can assist greatly by reassuring the patient.

Colonoscopy is used mainly for investigation purposes to detect a possible carcinoma, polyposis or ulcerative colitis, and enables multiple biopsies to be taken for histology.

In cases of a single polyp being observed diathermy can be applied.

GLUCOSE TOLERANCE TEST

The patient is given no food after supper but may have water to drink.
The following morning:
1) The bladder is emptied. The urine is saved and a blood sample is taken.
2) The patient then drinks 50 gram of glucose dissolved in 150 to 200 ml of water.
3) A sample of blood is taken at $\frac{1}{2}$, 1, $1\frac{1}{2}$, 2 and 3 hours after the glucose has been taken.
4) Urine is collected at 1 and 2 hours.
   All specimens are labelled with the patient's name, ward, date and time of the specimen collection.

UREA CLEARANCE TEST

No special preparation is required, but the patient should stay in bed and drink two tumblerfuls of water, to maintain a high urine volume.

1) The patient empties his bladder and the urine is discarded.
2) An hour later he empties his bladder and all the urine is saved. It is labelled with the exact time of voiding. Five ml of blood is taken and put into an oxylate tube.

Special Tests

3) An hour later, the patient empties
and the specimen is saved and
before. All these specimens are
laboratory.

   N.B. The bladder need not be emptied at intervals of exactly 60 minutes, provided the exact time of voiding is noted and the time put on the labels.

TO SAVE A 24 HOUR SPECIMEN OF URINE

No preparation of the patient is necessary but the procedure should be explained to gain his full co-operation.

At 8 am the bladder is emptied and the urine discarded. All subsequent urine voided should be placed in a Winchester, labelled with the patient's name, age, ward, at what time the collection commenced (8 am), and the appropriate date, to 8 am 24 hours later (date required). The last urine to be voided should be at the time stated on the label and placed in the bottle.

Various tests require dark Winchesters, or ones containing a preservative solution. These are usually obtained from the laboratory.

Special Tests

NORMAL RESULTS OF INVESTIGATIONS AND TESTS

Fasting blood sugar	3·3 to 5·5 millimole per litre of blood
Blood urea	2·5 to 7·5 millimole per litre of blood
Blood uric acid	0·20 to 0·43 millimole per litre of blood
Blood creatinine	50 to 130 micromole per litre of blood
Serum calcium	2·10 to 2·60 millimole per litre of blood
Haemoglobin	145 grams per litre of blood
Red cells	4·5 to 5·5 million per cubic millimetre
Blood sedimentation rate	Men 1 to 9 millimetres per hour
	Women 1 to 14 millimetres per hour
Bleeding time	2–7 minutes
Coagulation time	1–2 minutes
Prothrombin time	10–12 seconds
Urea clearance	75 per cent
Cerebrospinal fluid pressure	−5 to +5 mm of water
Pentagastrin test meal	Basal Acid Output 1 to 8 millimole per hour
	Peak Acid Output 1 to 50 millimole per hour

Incubation Periods of Infectious Diseases

Disease	Incubation Period	Period of Isolation
Chickenpox (Varicella)	7–23 days	Until last scab has separated
Diphtheria	1–6 days	Until 3 consecutive nose and throat swabs are negative
German Measles (Rubella)	17–18 days	Seven days from appearance of rash
Influenza	1–3 days	Up to 7 days
Measles (Morbilli)	10–14 days	Fourteen days from appearance of rash
Mumps (Infective Parotitis)	7–23 days	One week after swelling has subsided
Poliomyelitis	7–14 days	Usually 3 weeks

Disease	Incubation Period	Period of Isolation
Scarlet Fever (Scarlatina)	1–3 days	At least four weeks from appearance of rash
Smallpox (Variola)	12–14 days	Until every scab has separated
Salmonella	6–48 hours	Until 3 consecutive stools are negative
Sonne Dysentery	A few hours –2 days	Until 3–6 faecal specimens are negative
Typhoid Fever	12–14 days	Until 3 specimens of urine and faeces are negative
Whooping Cough (Pertussis)	7–14 days	3 to 4 weeks
Lassar Fever	3–17 days	Until absence of virus in urine
Rabies	2–6 weeks, can be up to 9 months	Until death occurs

Index

Abbreviations, Latin, 95
Abdomen, tapping the, 78
Abscess, opening an, 77
Act, Controlled Drugs, 91
  Pharmacy 1971, 91–4
  Poisons and Pharmacy, 1933, 93
Acupuncture, 65
Airways, 17
Albuminometer, 29
Anaesthetic,
  intravenous, pentothal, 71
Analgesic, local, 65
Aneurysm needle, 18
Antrum puncture, 66
  trocar and cannula for, 13
Apparatus for, continuous bladder irrigation, 27
  decompression of the bladder, 26
  intravenous fluids, 21
  peritoneal dialysis, 18
  rectal infusion, 24
  vaginal douche, 31
Artificial feeding, gastrostomy, 48
  oesophageal, 48
Aseptic techniques, 65–83
Aural dressing forceps, 17
  syringe, 13
  speculum, 30

Baby, bathing a, 41
Baths, medicated, 42
  temperature of, 42
Bed, bathing in, 40
Bililabstix, 102
Bladder lavage, 69
  syringe, 13
Blood culture, 74
  donor, 74
  grouping, 75
  pressure, est. of, 107
  transfusion, 72

Cannulae, butterfly, 23; Venflon, 23
Catheterization, female, 66
  male, 67
Catheters, various, 25
Central venous pressure, 73
Cervical smear, 63
Chest, aspiration of, 80
Colonoscopy, 108
Connections, graduated plastic, 14
Continuous bladder drainage, 68

Disinfection, methods of, 38
Douche, vaginal, 62
Dressings, simple, 75
  removal of clips, 76
  removal of sutures, 76

Ear, examination of, 46
  syringing, 46
Enema, purgative, 58
Energy, daily requirements, 98
  food yields, 98
Examination of ear, nose and throat, 46
Eye, application of ointment, 45
  instillation of drops, 45
  irrigation, 44
  rod, 32

Flatus tube, passing a, 59
Food values, 97
Forceps, various, 15–16

Glucose tolerance test, 110

Hair, combing of verminous, 44
  washing in bed, 43
Head mirror, 34
Higginson's syringe, 13

Ice bag, 56
  poultice, 56
Illustrations, 13–33
Incontinent patient, care of the, 42
Incubation periods, 113
Infectious diseases, 113
Infusions, cut down, 73
  intravenous, 72
  subcutaneous, 75
Injections, hypodermic, 70
  intramuscular, 70
  serum, 71
Instruments, illustrations, 15–18
Intravenous cannulae, 23
Intravenous pentothal, 71
Irrigation, of eye, 44

Index

Isolation periods, 113

Kaolin poultice, 55

Lavage, bladder, 69
  colonic, 59
  gastric, 51
  rectal, 59
Lotions, dilutions of, 89
Lumbar puncture, 78

Manometer, 19
Maxwell box, 22
M.C. oxygen mask, 20
Medicines, administration of, 52
Metric measures, 84
Mouth, care of, 43
  gags, 16

Nasal speculum, 30
Needles, aneurysm, 18
  disposable, 14
  lumbar puncture, 19
Neurological examination, 53
Nose, examination of, 32

Oesophageal feeds, nasal route, 49
  oral route, 48
  tube for, 28
Oxygen, administration of, 53
  apparatus for, 20–1
  tent, 54

Paracentesis abdominis, 78
Paracentesis thoracis, 80
Peritoneal dialysis, 79
  apparatus, 18
Pessaries, illustrations, 31
  insertion of, 64
Plaster of Paris, application of, 54
  removal, 54
Pneumothorax, aspiration of, 81
Poultices, ice, 56
  kaolin, 55
  starch, 57
Preparation for treatment, 35
Probe, 17
Proctoscope, 31

Quinsy, opening of, 47

Rectal, examination, 57
  lavage, 59
Roberts' trocar and cannula, 19
Ryle's duodenal tube, 28

Scalpel, Bard Parker, 32
Senoran's evacuator, 28
Sigmoidoscopy, 57

Skin, shaving, 60
    traction, 60
Speculae, various, 30
Steam inhalation, 61
Sterilization methods, 37
Subcutaneous infusion, 75
Sutures, removal of, 76
Suturing a wound, 77
Syringes, various, 13–14

Temperature, pulse, and respiration, 40
Tepid sponging, 61
Test meal, 50
Tests,
    glucose tolerance, 110
    urea clearance, 110
    normal results of, 112
Thermometers, various, 29
Thermometric equivalents, 87
Throat, examination of, 46
    spatula, 32
    swab, 47
Tracheotomy, 82
    dilator, 34
    hook, 34
    nursing care of, 83
    retractor, 34
    tubes, 32
Trocar and cannulae,
    Lichtwitz antral, 13
    Roberts', 19
Tubes, various, 28

Undine, 32
Urea, clearance test, 110
Urine, clean specimen, 69
    mid-stream specimen, 70
    testing, 84
    twenty-four hour specimen, 111

Vaginal, examination, 63
    douche, 62
    high swab, 62
Ventimask, 21

Wallace nasal cannulae, 21

Weights, Apothecaries, 84
    metric in S.I. units, 84–8